I0101681

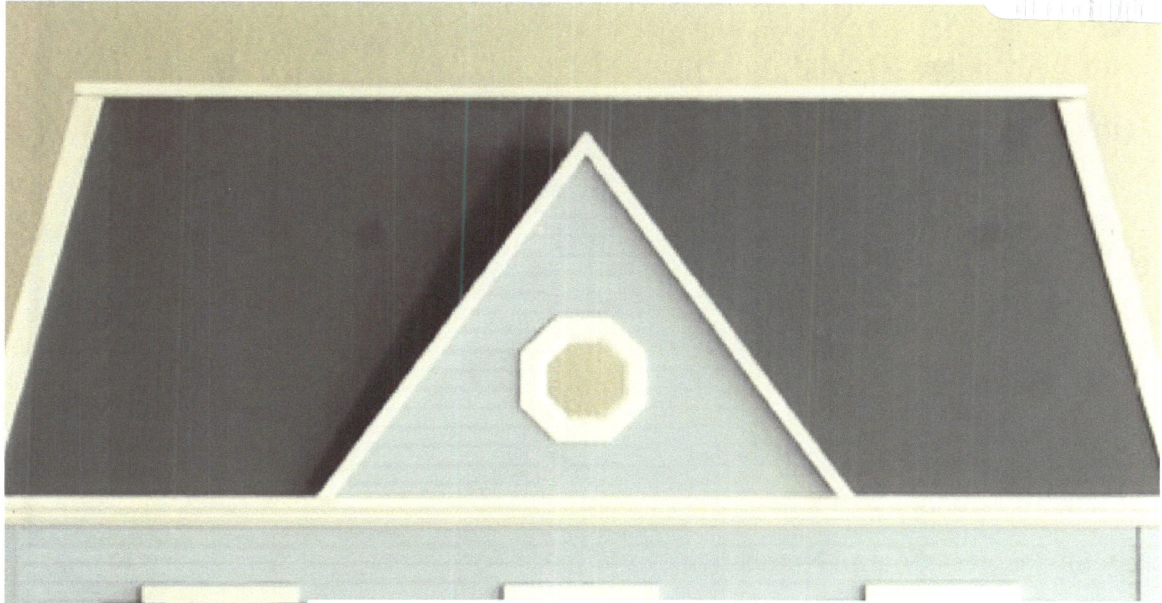

MARGARET WACKER, PH.D

MEMORY LANE

PHOTO PROMPTS TO TRIGGER MEMORIES

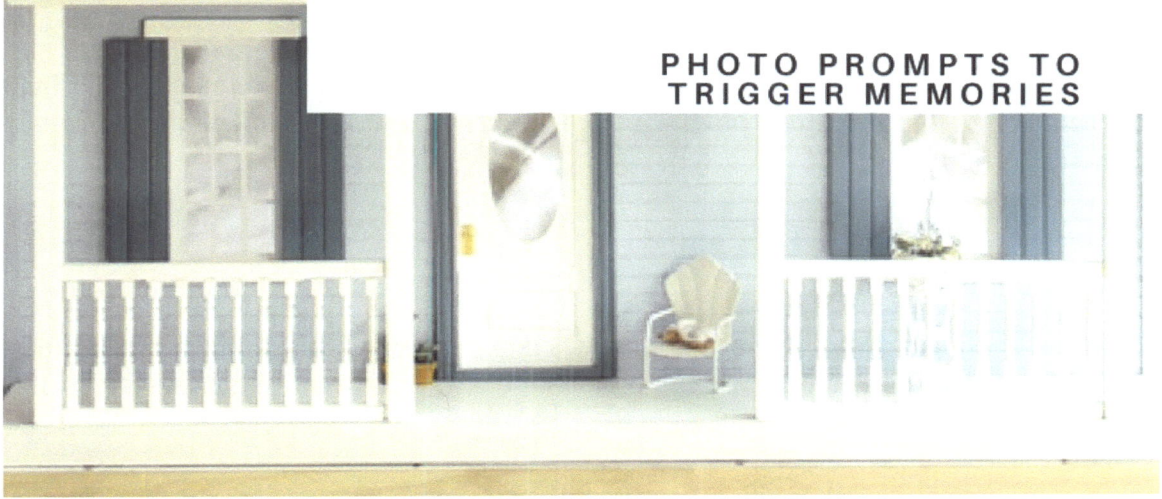

Memory Lane: Photo Prompts to Trigger Memories

By Margaret Wacker, Ph.D

Newhouse Creative Group

Orlando, Florida

www.NewhouseCreativeGroup.com

Copyright 2017, Margaret Wacker

Library of Congress Control Number: 2018947956

ISBN: 978-1-945493-06-5

Memory Lane: Photo Prompts to Trigger Memories by Margaret Wacker, Ph.D

Summary: Memory Lane uses photo prompts to 'trigger' memories. Structured questions built around common dollhouse objects prompt guided discussion and shared memories through group and paired interactions.

All rights reserved. No part of the material protected by this copyright may be reproduced or utilized in any form by any means without permission in writing from the copyright owner.

Introduction

Memory Lane uses photo prompts to 'trigger' memories. Structured questions built around common dollhouse objects prompt guided discussion and shared memories through group and paired interactions.

Why a Dollhouse?

A dollhouse brings memories to life.

In working with seniors over the years, I was amazed to see how certain stimuli, especially physical items, triggered their memories. When I used a dollhouse to test this approach, they shared their memories with great enthusiasm.

The various items in the dollhouse brought back memories and sparked conversations that were fun and delightful. That is what focusing on these items in a positive, open environment does. It encourages the sharing of memories. The seniors enjoyed these sessions and now you will, too.

Directions

Each unit in Memory Lane is focused on a specific room. Within the unit, you may want to spend more time on specific items in the room that spark more interest. It may be beneficial to make each individual item its own session or you may want to include all items from a room in one session. It's up to you to choose an optimal approach.

Whichever approach you choose, I've included the following to make the process as easy as possible for you.

- **Action** – Actions are printed in Italics and will say Action before them. These are actions to take during the session.
- **Discussion** – Along with the action, you will find a statement introducing the session as well as a number of prompts to stimulate the memory.
- **Notes** – These are tips to get the most out of this tool.

Special Thank You

A special thank you to my friend and editor, Mark H. Newhouse for his kindness and expertise.

Thanks also to my friends at Writers4Kids who have so generously offered their ideas and support.

This would not have been possible without the great photography of Taylor Lockwood and Stephanie Kondo, whose amazing dollhouses and enthusiastic support kept me excited.

I also need to thank Barbara Lipovics, who took my random notes and miraculously typed them up for me.

Thanks finally to everyone who shows so much love and caring for our seniors. This book is for them and you. I hope you find it enjoyable and helpful.

- Maggie

NOTE: You do not have to be a professional to enjoy sharing these materials and the conversations they trigger, just a caring person who loves sharing time with others.

Unit 1: The Dollhouse

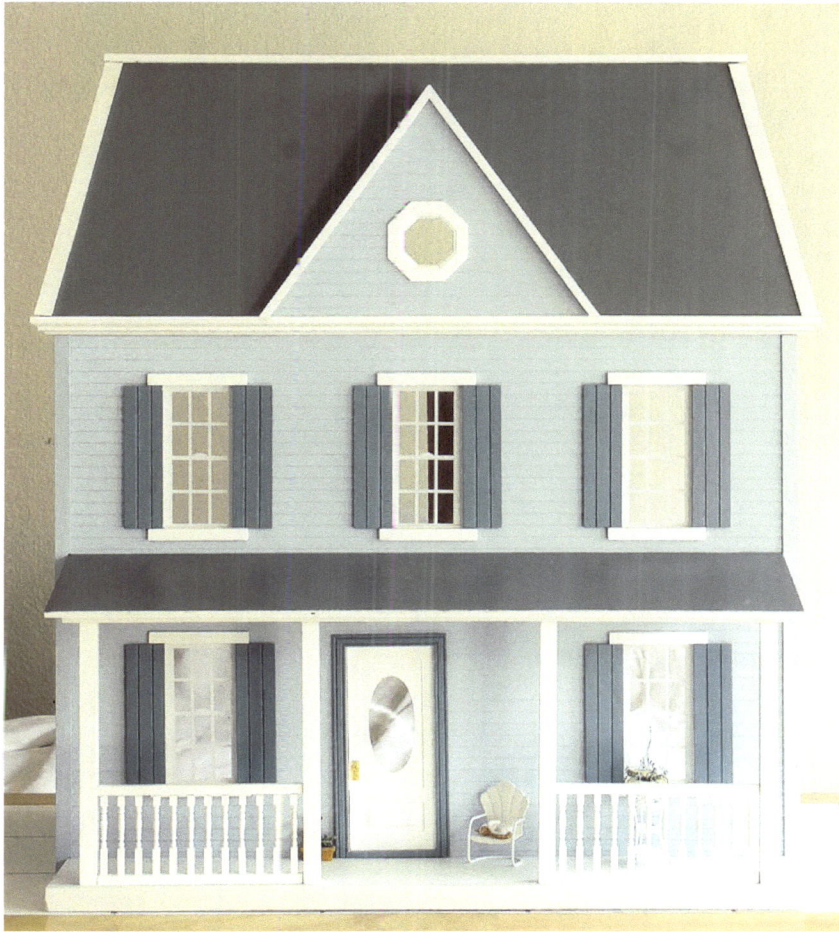

Action: *Present the dollhouse.*

People live in all kinds of houses: teepees, igloos, log cabins, etc.

- What kind of house did you live in?
- How many rooms did your house have?
- Where did you live?
- What is your favorite memory of life in your house?

Note: Even though the units are numbered, you do not have to follow the order given. You may select any room to start or ask if there is any room where they would like to start.

Unit 2: The Kitchen

The Sink

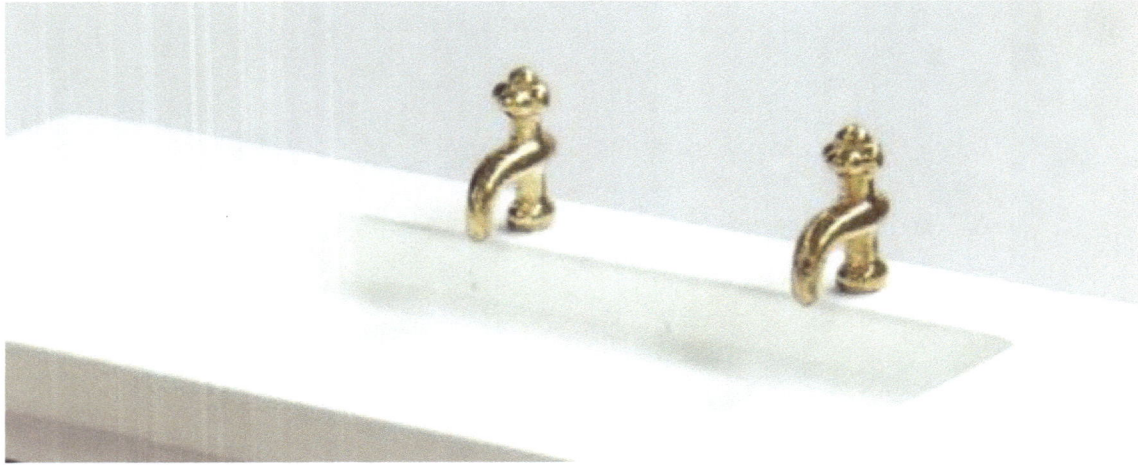

Action: *Present the sink.*

Every house has a kitchen. Every kitchen has a sink.

- What is your favorite memory that took place in the kitchen?
- What kind of kitchen sink did you have? What was it made of? What color was it?
- Was it difficult to get hot water? Do you remember heating a kettle on the stove for hot water?
- Did you help wash the dishes?
- Do you remember jelly glasses with television characters? Which did you have? Do you still have any?
- Did you ever wash your dog in the sink? What else did you do in the sink?
- Did you ever clean fish in the sink?
- What kind of soaps and detergents did you use?
- Do you remember the ads, slogans, or jingles for any of these products?
- When did you get your first dishwasher? What did you think when you first saw it?
- Did you ever bathe a baby in the sink? What do you remember about that?
- Did you ever have to pump water? What was that like?
- What else did you do in the sink?

The Stove/Range

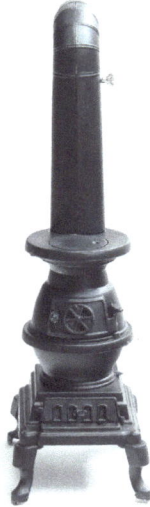

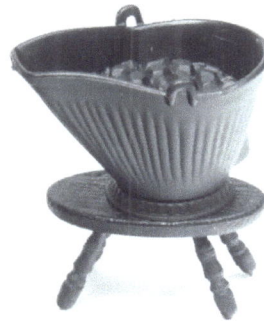

Action: *Present the stove/range.*

Every kitchen has a stove.

- What kind of stove did you have in your house?
- Did you ever have a potbelly stove?
- What kind of fuel did you use?
- Were there any safety rules about the stove?
- Who did the cooking in your family?
- What were some things they cooked?
- What was your favorite? Did you cook?
- How did you learn?
- Did anyone have a pet that slept near the stove?
- What other memories do you have about the kitchen?
- Was it the center of your family life?
- Can you describe their first stove (range)?

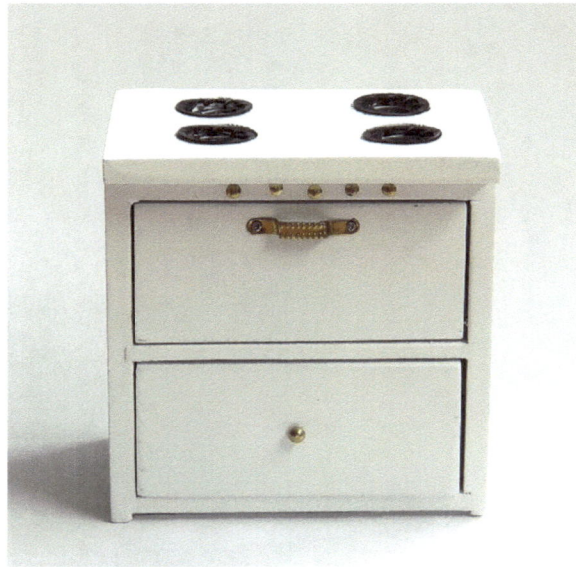

- What smells do you remember from home-cooked meals?
- What was your favorite meal?
- What was your least favorite food?
- How did your parents get you to eat?
- Did anyone help with the cooking? Did you?
- How did stoves change?
- How did foods you cook change? Remember TV dinners?
- How long did it take to make meals?
- Who did most of the cooking?
- What were special days for meals? Sundays? Holidays?
- What was your favorite place to get recipes?
- Who taught you to cook?
- What was the most unusual food you ever made?
- Was there a meal your family hated?
- What tricks do you know to get kids to eat certain foods? Remember Popeye and spinach?

The Icebox/Refrigerator

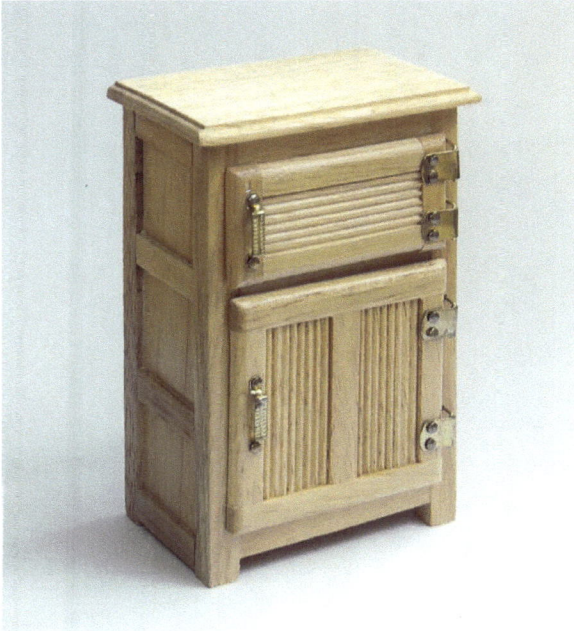

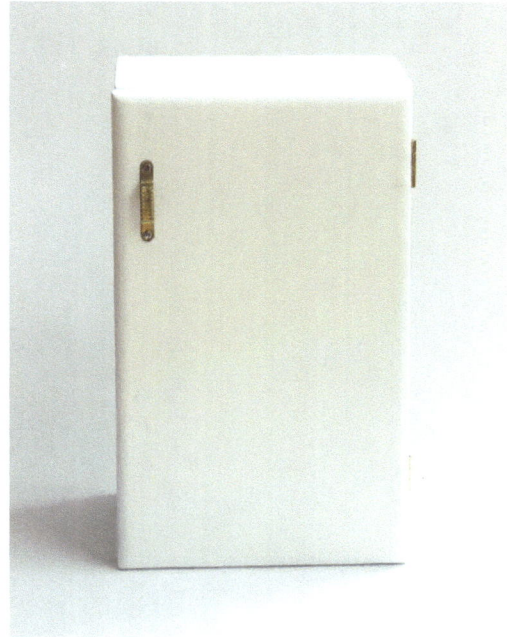

Action: *Present the Icebox/Refrigerator.*

Every kitchen has something to keep food cold.

- Did you ever have an icebox?
- How did you keep your food cold?
- Do you recall any problems with the icebox? Ordering the ice block? Emptying the drip pan?
- What was the smell like when you opened the door?
- How did keeping food cold change over the years?
- Do you remember your first refrigerator and how simple it was?
- Today's refrigerators have ice makers, crispers, cold water dispensers. Do you think these are good changes?

The Kitchen Table

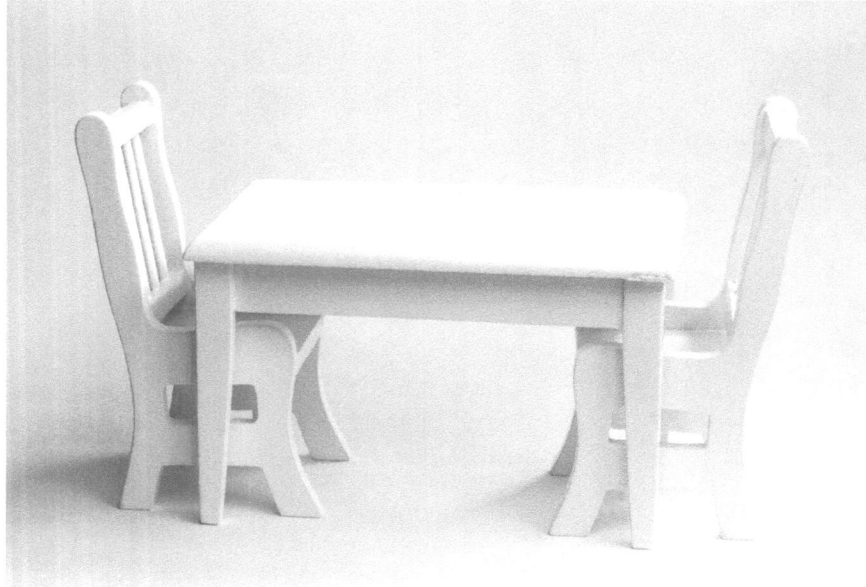

Action: *Present the kitchen table and chairs.*

Every kitchen has somewhere to eat.

- What kind of table and chairs did you have in your kitchen?
- Was the table round or square?
- Were there cushions on the chair?
- Did you have special seating like where you mom and dad always sat?
- Aside from eating, what other things did you do at the kitchen table? Did you do your homework there? Wrap gifts? Play with puzzles or games?
- Where did you get your first kitchen set? Did you ever make one?
- What lighting did you have for your kitchen?
- Why was the kitchen a favorite place for families to sit around? How has that changed?
- Did you have family meetings? What were they like? Who led them? How has that changed?
- What clothes did people wear to their meals when you were young? How did that change?
- What table coverings did you have?
- What floor covering did you have in the kitchen?
- How did radio and television change life around meals?

Unit 3: The Living Room

Let's check out the living room.

Do you have any memories about your living room?

What was your favorite place to sit and relax in your house and why?

The Fireplace

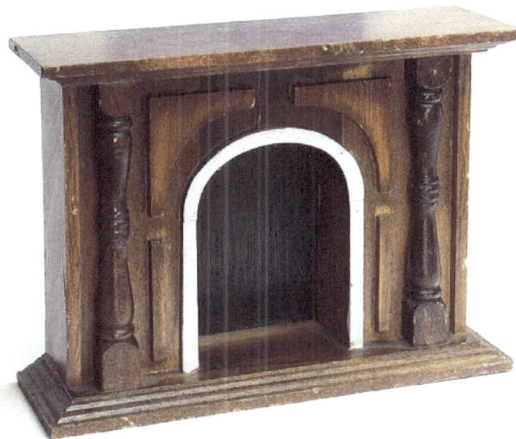

Action: *Present the fireplace.*

Some living rooms have fireplaces.

- Did you have a fireplace?
- What kind of fuel did you use? Coal? Wood?
- Did you hang stockings on the mantle at Christmas time?
- Did you have a hearth by your fireplace? Who slept on it? Your dog? Your cat?
- What was your favorite thing about spending time around the fireplace?
- What do you think about electric fireplaces?

Living Room Seating

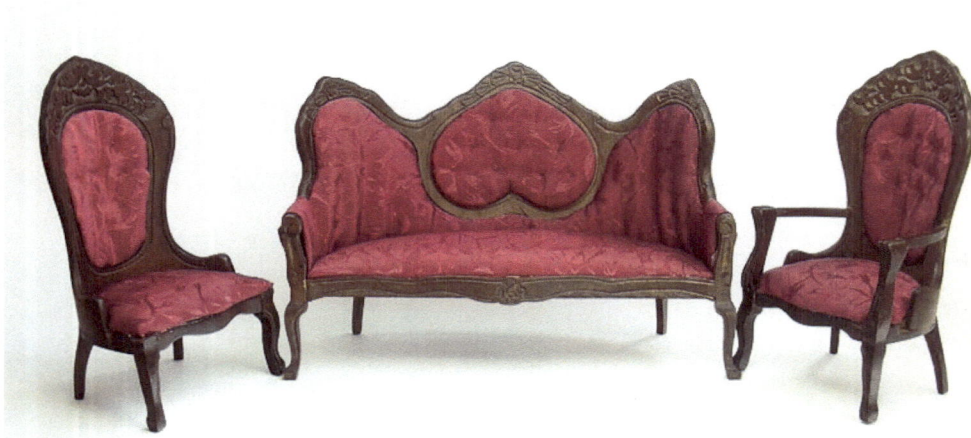

Action: *Present the couch and chairs.*

Every living room has somewhere to sit.

- What was in your living room?
- Was there a couch?
- Were there chairs?
- Were they comfortable? Did they have cushions?
- Did your mom and dad have special seats?
- Did you have plastic covers or doilies on the furniture?
- Where did your parents get their furniture from? Homemade? Stores?
- Did you have to keep pets off the furniture?

The Coffee Table

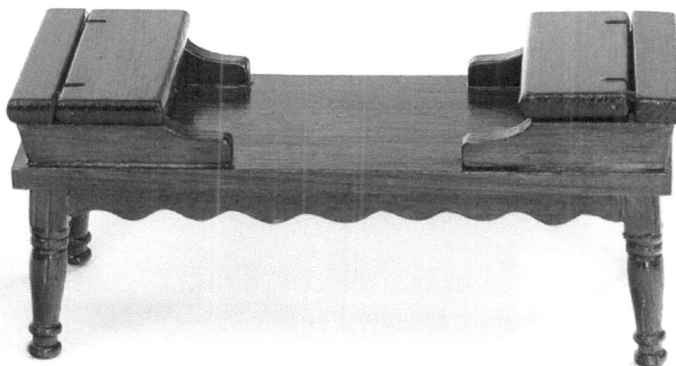

Action: *Present the coffee table.*

Some living rooms have coffee tables.

- Did you have a coffee table in the living room?
- What did you use it for?
- Was anyone allowed to put their feet up on it?
- Where did you get if from? Did someone make it?
- What are some things you kept on the table? Photos? TV Guide? Magazines?
- Did you have ashtrays? Who smoked? Did you smoke? How did you start? How did you stop?
- Did you have end tables? What were they like?

Unit 4: The Bathroom

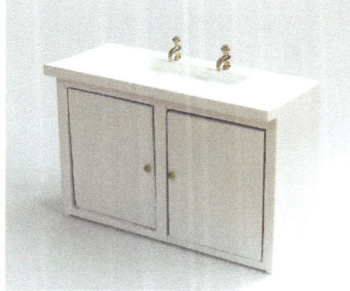

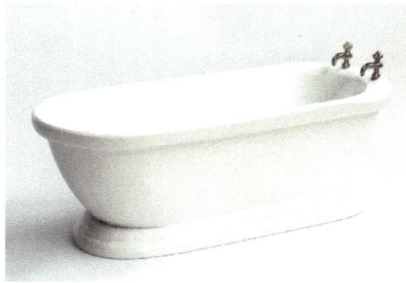

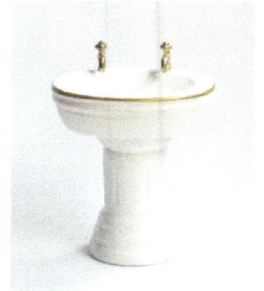

Action: *Present the bathroom (could include the sink, tub, and/or toilet).*

Every house today has at least one bathroom.

- How many bathrooms did you have?
- How did you manage if you only had one?
- What do remember about your bathroom?
- Can you describe the plumbing?
- Did ever have an overhead water tank that you pulled with a chain?
- What kind of bathtub did you have?
- Did you prefer showers or a bath?
- What wall coverings did you have?
- What personal products did you have?
- What perfumes or colognes did you use on your first date?
- What do you think of today's bathrooms with garden tubs, soaking tubs, Jacuzzis, built in showers, and bidets?
- What are some other things you had in your bathroom?
- Did you ever have an outhouse?
- Were you ever in the military and remember the 'fun' of digging a latrine?

Unit 5: The Bedroom

Every house has at least one bedroom. Usually you will find 2 or 3 bedrooms in a house, but some will have more.

- What do you remember about your bedroom?
- Did you have your own room or did you share?
- Who did you share with?
- Did you have shelves? What was on them? Books? Trophies? Baseball cards?
- What was on your walls? Photos? Posters? Placques?
- What was your closet like? Neat? Messy?
- What was in the closet that was special to you? Sports equipment, uniforms, baseball caps?
- Did you have a uniform in your closet from belonging to a group? Did you belong to a sports team? Scouts? Other groups and clubs?

The Bed

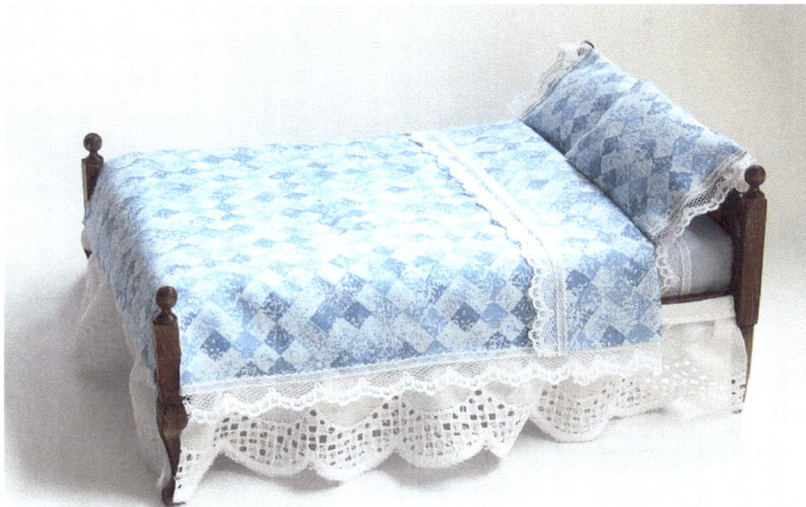

Action: *Present the bed.*

Every bedroom has a bed.

- Do you remember your bedspread or quilt?
- Did you keep your toys in your bedroom? Stuffed animals?

The Dresser

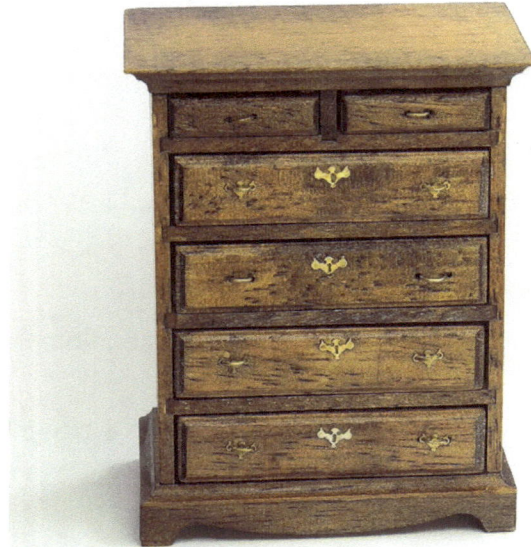

Action: *Present the dresser.*

Most bedrooms have a dresser to store things.

- What sorts of things did you keep in your dresser?
- Did any of the drawers have a lock? What would you keep in there?
- What was on top of your dresser?
- What was that special something you kept hidden in your dresser or room?
- Did you have a diary or journal? Do you still have it?
- What photographs were in your room?
- What did your lamp look like?
- What hobbies did you have?
- How were your clothes different from today?
- Did your mother make your clothes or shop for them?

Unit 6: Entertainment

The TV

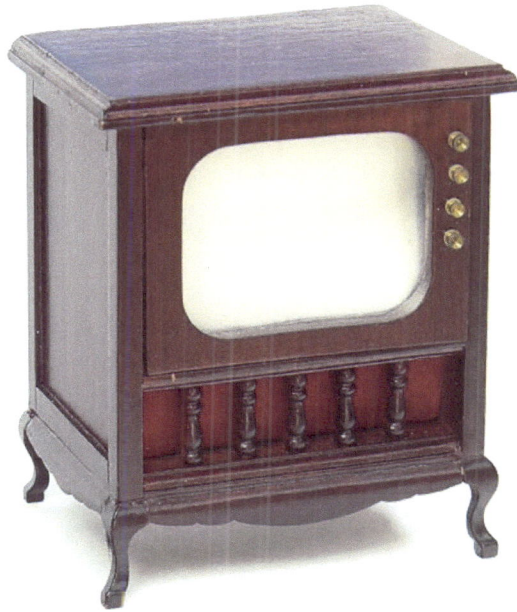

Action: *Present the TV.*

Some families watch TV for entertainment.

- When did you get your first TV?
- What did it look like?
- Did you ever have TV dinners?
- How did you get reception? Aluminum foil? Antenna? Rabbit ears?
- In what room did you watch TV? Did you have more than 1?
- What were your favorite TV shows?
- Do you remember any theme songs? Roy Rogers? Howdy Doody? Gene Autry?
- Can you sing any theme songs?
- Who were your favorite stars?
- What was the worst show on television? Why?

- How has TV changed since you were a child? What do you think of Large screens, remote controls, cable contracts, satellites, pay-per-view, VHS tapes, DVDs,, 24 hour news? Do you think these were good changes?
- What is the most important news story you remember watching on TV? Do you remember the lunar landing, the assassination of JFK and Martin Luther King, Queen Elizabeth's coronation, or Princes Diana's wedding? What else do you remember?
- Did you spend more time watching TV or reading books? Who were your favorite authors?

The Radio

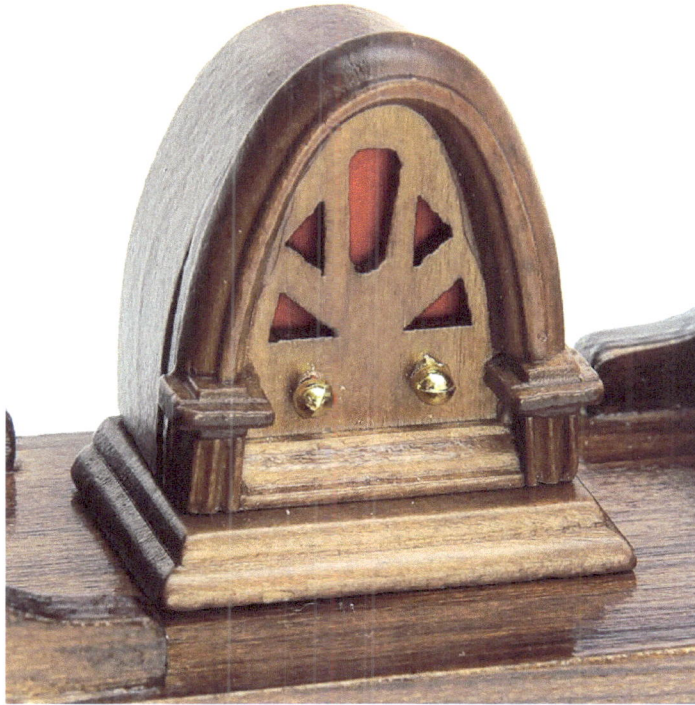

Action: *Present the radio.*

Many families used to listen to radios.

- Where was the radio kept in your house?
- What were your favorite radio programs?
- Do you remember the broadcasting of a major news event?
- What was that news?
- Where were you when you first heard the news?
- How has radio changed today? What do you think of pay radio like SiriusXM? Do you know about podcasts? Are these good changes?

The Record Player

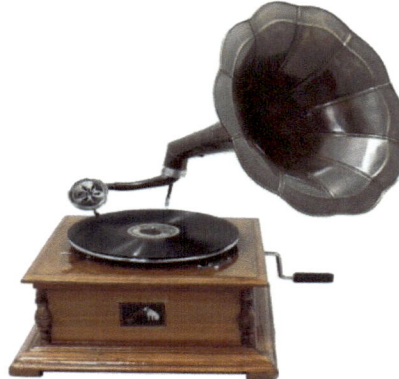

Action: *Present the record player.*

Some families used to listen to a record player.

- What kind of record player did you have? Hi-fi? Stereo?
- What kind of records did you listen to? Music? Comedy albums? Language records?
- What was your favorite music?
- Did you sing, dance, or play an instrument?
- Did you ever meet a celebrity? Singer? Actor?
- Did you go to concerts? Which ones do you remember?
- Did you know anyone who became a celebrity?
- Did you dream of becoming a star?
- Would you want to be a star now? Why? Why not?
- If you could invite a celebrity to dinner, who would it be?
- What are the biggest differences between the stars of yesterday and those of today?
- How do you feel about the way entertainment has changed from the day of the old record players to today?

Unit 7: The Front Porch

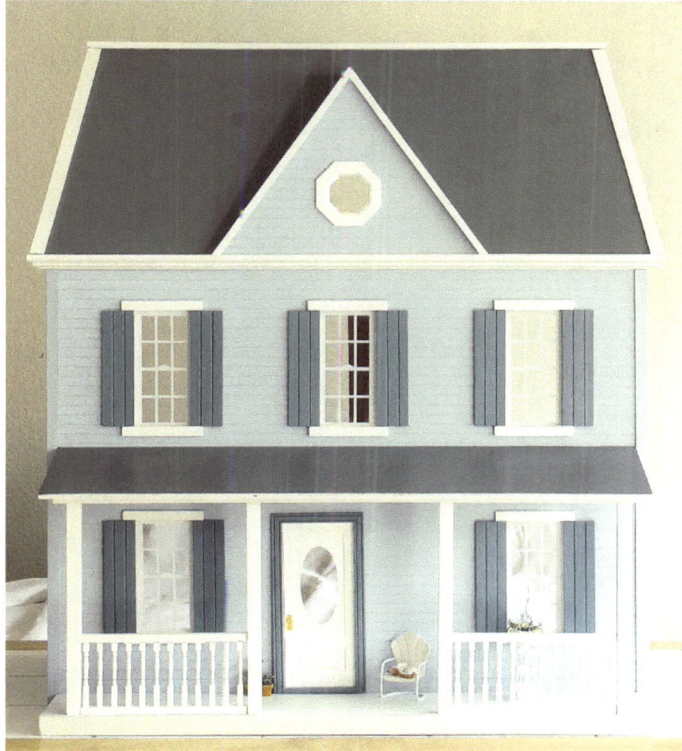

Action: *Present the dollhouse and point out the front porch.*

Many houses have a front porch.

- Did you have a front porch?
- What are your favorite memories about the front porch?
- Did your porch have a front swing? Rocking chair?
- Did neighbors stop by and visit you on the porch?
- Did you decorate the porch for holidays?
- What kind of decorations did you have?
- How was your porch different than a patio, terrace, or lanai?
- Did you have a back porch?

Unit 8: The Attic

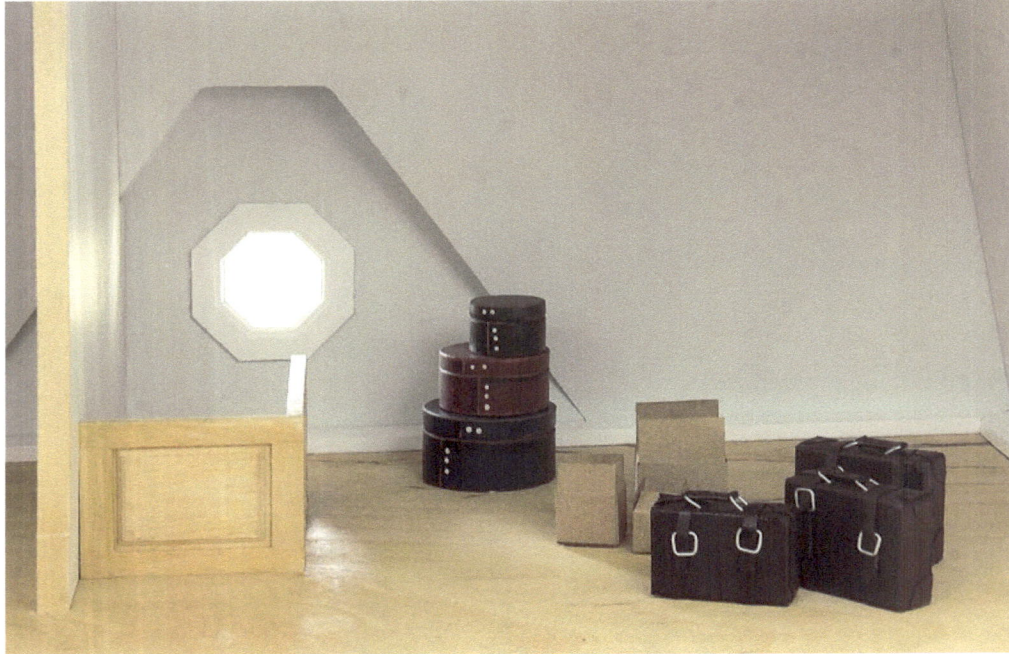

Action: *Present the attic.*

Some houses have an attic.

- Do you remember having an attic?
- Was it finished or unfinished?
- What kinds of things did you store there?
- Was it a scary place?
- What was different about it?
- Were there any secrets about the attic?
- What has changed about attics today? Is this a good change?
- What was the strangest thing stored in your attic?
- What was the oldest thing in your attic? In your house?

Unit 9: The Cellar/Basement

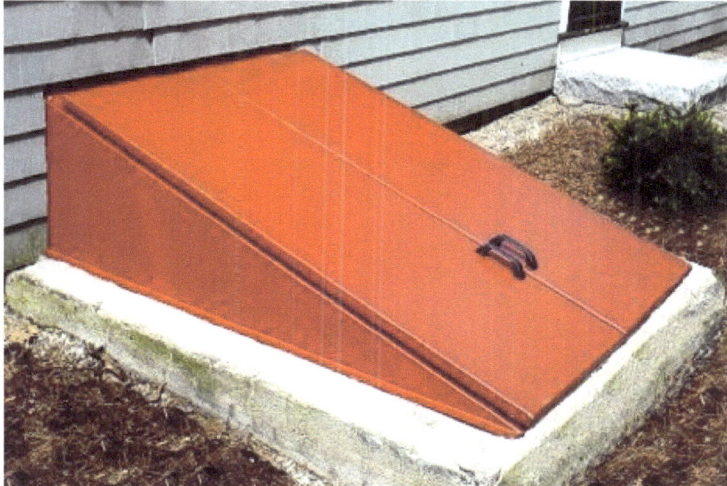

Action: *Show picture of cellar.*

Some houses have a cellar or basement.

- Did you have a cellar or basement in your house?
- What was kept there?
- Was it scary? Did you decorate it for Halloween?
- Was it finished or unfinished?
- Who finished your basement?
- What wall covering was there? Paneling?
- What did you do down there? Parties?
- What hobbies did you have? Did you have a dark room, pool table, ping pong table?
- Did you have toy trains? Car racing set?
- What furniture did you have?
- Name something about your basement for each of the 5 senses: touch, smell, vision, hearing, taste.
- How have basements changed?

Unit 10: The Garage

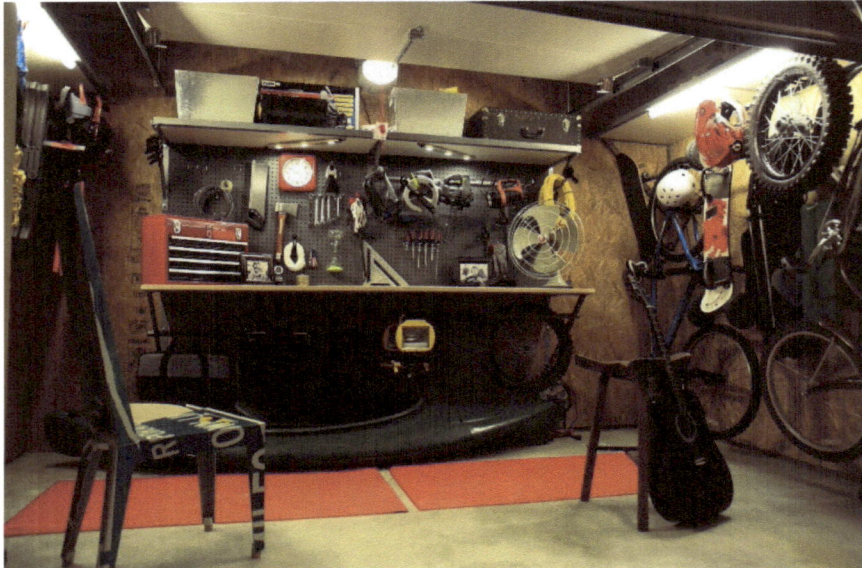

Some houses have a garage.

- Did you have a garage?
- Where was it located? Was it attached or free-standing?
- Was your garage a mess or neat? How was it organized?
- What did you keep in the garage? Cars? Tools? Lawn mower? Lawn furniture? Bicycles? Boat, Motorcycles? Golf clubs?
- What funny stories do you have about the items in your garage?
- Did you ever play in the garage? What kinds of playing did you do in the garage? Hop scotch? Hide-and-seek?
- What other activities happened in your garage? Parties?
- What was your first car? How have cars changed?
- What kind of changes are there in garages today? Automatic door openers? Larger car spaces? Are these good changes?
- What was your driveway like?
- What was on your driveway? Cars? R.V.s?
- If you had an R.V., what was your fondest memory? What was your funniest disaster?

Thank You

I want to thank you for all the work you do helping others capture their memories. I hope this book helps you. Remember, you can use as many objects as you like, not just the ones here, to help trigger the wonderful memories people love sharing.

I think the most important advice I can give you is to have fun and then those you work with will have fun too. I've loved working with seniors and hope you will send me your ideas and comments by visiting my website at MemoryLane.NewhouseCreativeGroup.com

Supplementary Materials Available

If you like this guide, you can order other materials to supplement it. We offer:

- Memory Lane Photo Pack - Blow-up photos of the objects depicted in this book with questions on the reverse.
- Our Stories - A template for producing a book of your friends' memories aligned with this book.
- Memory Lane for Men - Prompts to stir the memory of men.

All are either available now or coming soon in soft cover or eBook and can be purchased on Amazon or from NewhouseCreativeGroup.com. Ask about group discounts.

Want a Dollhouse?

While we've used high quality photos of a dollhouse and the objects within to help you spark memories, having a real dollhouse may produce even greater results.

You can search online to purchase a dollhouse or visit us online at MemoryLane.NewhouseCreativeGroup.com for suggestions of dollhouse retailers.

Share Your Experience

We appreciate your work so much and hope your experience was enjoyable. We invite you to share your thoughts and help us improve future editions of our memory triggering program by taking a short survey at MemoryLane.NewhouseCreativeGroup.com.

Annotated Bibliography

Reminiscence and Older People Health

Coleman, P.T. *Uses of Reminiscence: Functions and benefits.* Aging & mental health, July (2005), 9(4):291-294. This is an early work that notes that thirty to forty years ago, reminiscence was associated with senility. Now it is a popular approach to improving older people's mental health.

Reminiscence in Long-Term Care

Cooney, A., Hunter, A., Murphy, K.,Dympna, C., et al.

Seeing Me Through My Memories: Grounded Theory Study On Using Reminiscence With People With Dementia Living in Long-Term Care. Journal of Critical Nursing, (2014), 23 3564-3574. These authors noted that reminiscence enabled staff to see and know the person beneath the dementia. Knowing the person enabled the staff to understand and sometimes to accommodate the person's current behavior. As a result, they found that that reminiscence enhanced the experience of living in long-term care for residents with dementia and working in long-term care for staff.

Reminiscence as a Therapeutic Intervention

Gonzales, J., Mayordomo, T., Torres, M., Sales, A., Melendez, J.

Reminiscence and Dementia:a Therapeutic Intervention. International Psychogeriatrics, (2015), 27:10, 1731-1737. These authors examined the benefits of an integrative reminiscence program in elderly people with dementia. Their results supported a reduction in depression symptoms and improvement in psychological well-being. They also shared their experiences with optimal group size and number of sessions necessary to achieve their results.

Reminiscence and Prompts

Dempsey, L. Murphy , K., Cooney, A., Dympna, C. et al. *Reminiscence and Dementia: A Concept Analysis.* Dementia, (2014), vol. 12 (2) 176-192. These authors defined reminiscence in people with dementia as the deliberate use of prompts, for example, photographs, aromas, music, and questioning, to provide enjoyment and foster a sense of achievement and self-worth.

In addition, these authors addressed a frequent concern about the possibility of stimulating unhappy memories. They report that a study of naturally occurring reminiscences indicated that 67% of these unhappy reminiscences occurred as a result of negative emotions, primarily sadness or nostalgia. They suggest that by adopting a person-centered approach to patient care and having knowledge of the individual, potential problems should be avoided in these reminiscence sessions.

Meet the Author: Maggie Wacker

Margaret Wacker has been an advanced practice nurse for a lot of wonderful years. Her experience includes a wide range of specialty areas such as psychiatric nursing, family therapy, pain management, legal consulting, and academic positions at state and private colleges. For the past ten years she has helped families care for their loved ones with dementia. The use of dollhouse prompts evolved out of her desire to tap positive memories from the past in people who were memory challenged. She wants to help others benefit from her experience and hopes her work makes triggering memories simple and fun.

Visit wackerandassociates.com for more about Maggie and her professional career.

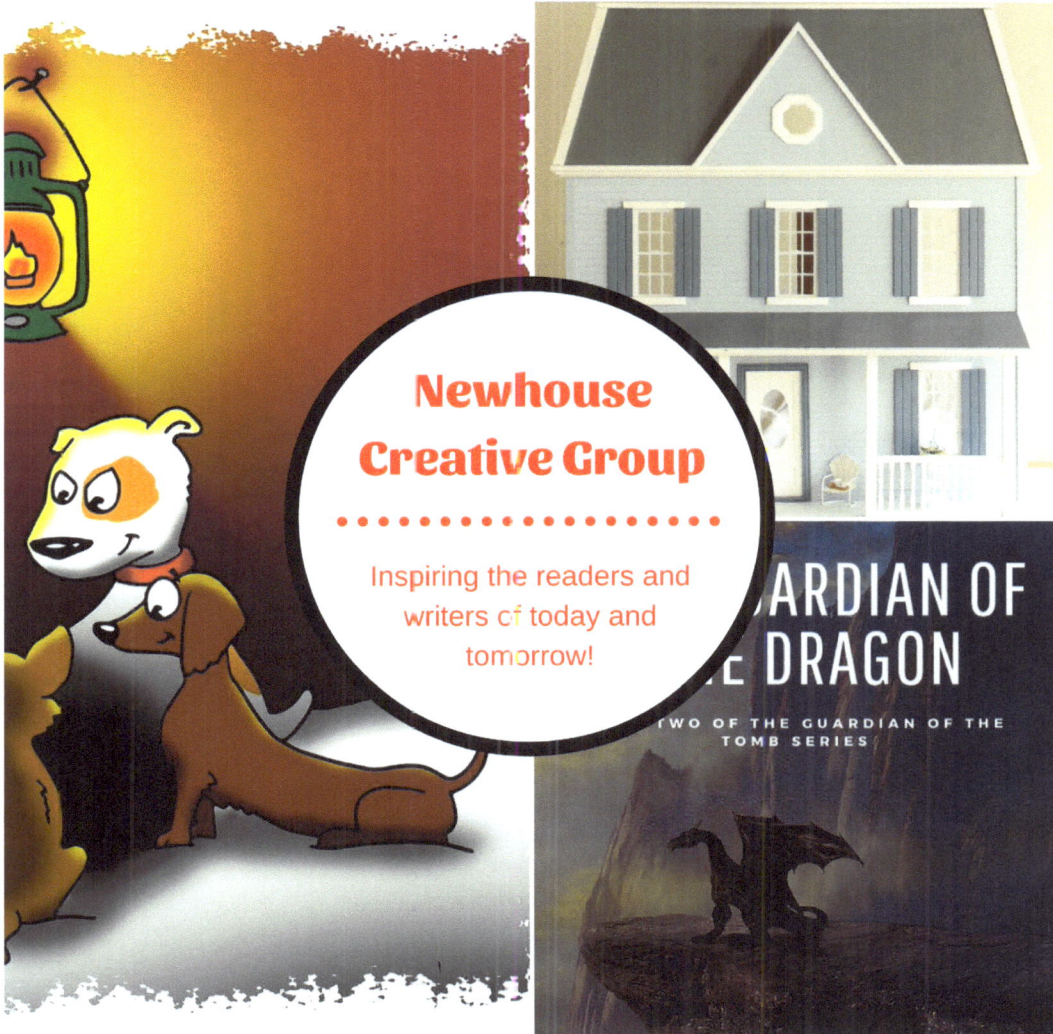

Newhouse Creative Group

· · · · · · · · · · · · · · · · · · · ·

Inspiring the readers and writers of today and tomorrow!

GUARDIAN OF THE DRAGON

TWO OF THE GUARDIAN OF THE TOMB SERIES

Visit NewhouseCreativeGroup.com for more books and other products from NCG Key, AimHi Press, and the rest of the Newhouse Creative Group family!

www.ingramcontent.com/pod-product-compliance
Lightning Source LLC
Chambersburg PA
CBHW060840270326
41933CB00002B/151